Sirtfood Diet Guide for Beginners

Understanding the Importance of Sirtfood Diet

By

Cormac Dairmid

Table of Contents

CHAPTER 1 6

Introduction 6

1.1 What is the Sirtfood Diet? 6

1.2 How Does the Sirtfood Diet Work? 7

CHAPTER 2 12

Sirtfoods: The Key Players..........12

2.1 What are Sirtfoods? 12

2.2 List of Common Sirtfoods..13

2.3 Understanding the Benefits 17

CHAPTER 3 21

The Science Behind Sirtuins 21

3.1 Sirtuins: The Molecular Heroes.....................................21

3.2 How Sirtuins Impact Your Health 24

3.3 Sirtuins and Weight Management 26

CHAPTER 4 29

Getting Started with the Sirtfood Diet 29

4.1 Preparing Mentally and Emotionally 29

4.2 Setting Realistic Goals 31

4.3 Creating a Meal Plan 33

CHAPTER 5 37

Phase 1: The Sirtfood Diet Jumpstart 37

5.1 The First 3 Days 37

5.2 Sample Meal Plan..............39

5.3 Tips for Success................40

CHAPTER 6 44

Phase 2: Maintenance and Sustainable Eating 44

6.1 Transitioning to Phase 2 45

6.2 Long-Term Sirtfood Eating 48

6.3 Recipe Ideas and Inspiration 52

CHAPTER 7 56

Sirtfood Diet and Weight Loss 56

7.1 How the Diet Supports Weight Loss 56

7.2 Realistic Expectations 61

7.3 Monitoring Progress 64

CHAPTER 8 68

Incorporating Exercise and Lifestyle Changes 68

8.1 The Role of Exercise 68

8.2 Stress Management and Sleep 71

8.3 Staying Active and Healthy 73

CHAPTER 9 77

Common Challenges and How to
Overcome Them 77

9.1 Dealing with Cravings 77

9.2 Social and Dining Out
Challenges 80

9.3 Plateau Busting Strategies .. 82

CHAPTER 1

Introduction

1.1 What is the Sirtfood Diet?

The Sirtfood Diet is a popular and relatively recent dietary regimen that has gained attention for its unique approach to weight management and overall health. At its core, the Sirtfood Diet is founded on the consumption of specific foods known as "Sirtfoods" that are rich in a group of proteins called sirtuins. These sirtuins, particularly SIRT1, play a pivotal role in regulating various cellular processes, including metabolism and inflammation. The diet's proponents argue that by increasing your intake of these Sirtfoods, you can activate your sirtuins, which, in turn, may help promote weight loss, improve metabolic health, and provide other potential health benefits.

1.2 How Does the Sirtfood Diet Work?

The Sirtfood Diet operates on the premise that by consuming foods rich in sirtuins, individuals can activate these proteins in their bodies. Sirtuins are enzymes that are involved in regulating various cellular processes, including DNA repair, inflammation control, and metabolism. They are often referred to as "longevity proteins" because of their potential role in promoting healthy aging and longevity.

Here's a simplified explanation of how the Sirtfood Diet works:

- **Phase 1: Sirtfood Diet Jumpstart**: The diet typically begins with a strict phase that lasts for a few days, often referred to as the "jumpstart" phase. During this period, calorie intake is significantly reduced, and individuals consume a limited selection of Sirtfoods. This phase is designed to kickstart the body's metabolism and promote weight loss.

- **Phase 2: Maintenance and Sustainable Eating**: After the initial phase, individuals transition into a more balanced and sustainable eating plan. They continue to include Sirtfoods in their daily meals but also introduce a wider variety of foods to ensure a balanced diet. This phase is intended for long-term adherence to the diet's principles.

- **Regular Consumption of Sirtfoods**: Throughout the diet, the emphasis is placed on regularly incorporating Sirtfoods into meals. Some of the commonly recommended Sirtfoods include kale, broccoli, green tea, extra-virgin olive oil, red wine, dark chocolate, and turmeric. These foods are believed to activate sirtuins and support overall health.

- **Calorie Restriction**: Caloric intake is controlled, particularly during the jumpstart phase, to create a calorie deficit that can facilitate weight loss. However, the diet promotes the consumption of nutrient-dense foods to ensure that individuals still receive essential nutrients despite reduced calorie intake.

- **Exercise**: The Sirtfood Diet encourages regular physical activity as part of a healthy lifestyle. Exercise complements the diet's goals by further enhancing metabolic function and promoting overall well-being.

Sirtfood Diet is centered around the concept of activating sirtuins through the consumption of Sirtfoods, with the ultimate aim of improving metabolic health and supporting weight loss. While it has gained attention for its unique approach, it's important for individuals considering this diet to consult with a healthcare professional to ensure it aligns with their specific health goals and needs. Additionally, research on the long-term effects of the Sirtfood Diet is still ongoing, and more evidence is needed to fully understand its potential benefits and limitations.

CHAPTER 2

Sirtfoods: The Key Players

2.1 What are Sirtfoods?

Sirtfoods are a category of foods that are rich in sirtuin-activating compounds. Sirtuins are a group of proteins, specifically SIRT1 through SIRT7, that play a crucial role in regulating various cellular processes. They are often associated with longevity, metabolic health, and overall well-being. Sirtfoods are believed to stimulate the activity of sirtuins, particularly SIRT1, which can have a positive impact on health.

These foods are characterized by their high content of polyphenolic compounds, particularly resveratrol, quercetin, and epicatechin, which are known to activate sirtuins. Sirtfoods are typically plant-based and are packed with essential nutrients, antioxidants, and other bioactive compounds that contribute to their potential health benefits.

2.2 List of Common Sirtfoods

Here is a list of some common Sirtfoods that are often recommended as part of the Sirtfood Diet:

1. **Kale:** Kale is often considered a superstar Sirtfood. It's packed with nutrients, including vitamins A, C, and K, as well as minerals like calcium and magnesium.

2. **Broccoli:** Broccoli is rich in sulforaphane, a compound that may have anti-inflammatory and anticancer properties.

3. **Green Tea:** Green tea contains epigallocatechin gallate (EGCG), a polyphenol known for its antioxidant properties. It's also believed to activate sirtuins.

4. **Extra-Virgin Olive Oil:** Rich in monounsaturated fats and antioxidants, olive oil is a staple in Mediterranean diets and is associated with various health benefits.

5. **Turmeric:** Curcumin, the active compound in turmeric, is known for its anti-inflammatory and antioxidant properties.

6. **Onions:** Onions contain quercetin, a flavonoid that may have anti-inflammatory and antiviral properties.

7. **Red Wine:** Red wine is a source of resveratrol, a polyphenol associated with cardiovascular health and longevity.

8. **Dark Chocolate (Cocoa):** Dark chocolate with a high cocoa content contains flavonoids like epicatechin, which may have heart-protective effects.

9. **Walnuts:** Walnuts are rich in omega-3 fatty acids and polyphenols, making them a heart-healthy choice.

10. **Strawberries:** Strawberries are a good source of quercetin and

vitamin C, which can support immune function.

11. **Buckwheat:** Buckwheat is a gluten-free grain that contains rutin, a flavonoid that may have antioxidant properties.

12. **Medjool Dates:** Dates are a natural source of nutrients and fiber, providing a natural sweetener for Sirtfood recipes.

13. **Arugula:** Arugula is a leafy green vegetable that is often included in salads and is rich in vitamins and minerals.

14. **Lovage:** Lovage is an herb that is used in culinary dishes and is known for its potential health benefits.

15. **Parsley:** Parsley is a herb that is rich in vitamins, particularly

vitamin K, and can be added to various dishes for flavor and nutrition.

2.3 Understanding the Benefits

The potential benefits of Sirtfoods are closely tied to their ability to activate sirtuins. When sirtuins are activated, they may contribute to the following health benefits:

- **Improved Metabolism:** Sirtuins play a role in regulating metabolism, including the breakdown of fats and the production of energy. Activating sirtuins may help enhance metabolic efficiency and potentially support weight management.

- **Anti-Inflammatory Effects:** Many Sirtfoods contain anti-inflammatory compounds, which can help reduce chronic inflammation, a key factor in various chronic diseases.

- **Cellular Repair and Longevity:** Sirtuins are associated with DNA repair and cellular maintenance, which may contribute to healthy aging and longevity.

- **Cardiovascular Health:** Some Sirtfoods, such as red wine and olive oil, are linked to heart health. They may help reduce the risk of cardiovascular diseases by promoting healthy blood pressure and cholesterol levels.

- **Antioxidant Protection:** Sirtfoods are often rich in antioxidants that help protect cells from oxidative stress and damage caused by free radicals.

- **Weight Management:** By improving metabolism and reducing inflammation, Sirtfoods may support weight loss and weight maintenance efforts.

It's important to note that while Sirtfoods offer potential health benefits, they are most effective when consumed as part of a balanced diet that includes a variety of nutrient-rich foods. Additionally, more research is needed to fully understand the extent of their health-promoting properties and their long-term effects. People interested in the Sirtfood Diet should consult with a healthcare professional or registered dietitian before making significant dietary changes to ensure that it aligns with their individual health goals and needs.

CHAPTER 3

The Science Behind Sirtuins

3.1 Sirtuins: The Molecular Heroes

Sirtuins, often referred to as "molecular heroes," are a family of proteins found in all living organisms, from bacteria to humans. These proteins play a critical role in regulating a wide range of cellular processes, making them essential for overall health and longevity.

There are seven sirtuins in mammals, known as SIRT1 through SIRT7, and they are primarily involved in maintaining the integrity of our cells and DNA. Sirtuins are often associated with the following key functions:

- **DNA Repair:** Sirtuins are involved in repairing damaged DNA, which is crucial for preventing mutations that can lead to cancer and other diseases. They help maintain genomic stability and integrity.

- **Cellular Metabolism:** Sirtuins play a central role in regulating metabolism by controlling the balance between energy production (catabolism) and storage (anabolism). They promote the breakdown of fats and carbohydrates for energy and help maintain energy homeostasis.

- **Inflammation Regulation:**
  Sirtuins have anti-inflammatory
  properties and can suppress
  pro-inflammatory signaling
  pathways. This helps reduce
  chronic inflammation, a factor
  in many chronic diseases.

- **Cell Survival:** Sirtuins can
  promote cell survival by
  preventing programmed cell
  death (apoptosis) in response to
  cellular stress. This is important
  for tissue repair and overall
  longevity.

- **Longevity:** Sirtuins are often
  associated with lifespan
  extension and promoting
  healthy aging in various
  organisms. Their activation has
  been shown to extend the
  lifespans of yeast, worms, flies,
  and mice in laboratory studies.

3.2 How Sirtuins Impact Your Health

The impact of sirtuins on health is profound and far-reaching. Here's how sirtuins can positively affect your overall well-being:

- **Aging and Longevity:** Research in various model organisms suggests that sirtuins may play a role in extending lifespan and promoting healthy aging. While the effects on human longevity are still being studied, their involvement in DNA repair and cellular maintenance makes them key players in the aging process.

- **Metabolic Health:** Sirtuins, particularly SIRT1, are heavily involved in regulating metabolism. They can enhance

insulin sensitivity, improve
glucose control, and promote
efficient energy utilization.
This makes them potential
targets for managing conditions
like type 2 diabetes and obesity.

- **Cardiovascular Health:**
  Sirtuins are associated with
  protecting the cardiovascular
  system. They can help reduce
  oxidative stress, lower blood
  pressure, and improve blood
  vessel function. These effects
  can lower the risk of heart
  disease.

- **Neurological Health:** Sirtuins
  may have neuroprotective
  properties. They are linked to
  improved brain function,
  cognitive function, and may
  play a role in preventing

neurodegenerative diseases like Alzheimer's and Parkinson's.

- **Inflammation Control:** Sirtuins' ability to suppress inflammation is significant. Chronic inflammation is a contributor to many diseases, including cancer, autoimmune disorders, and heart disease. Activating sirtuins can help mitigate inflammation.

3.3 Sirtuins and Weight Management

Sirtuins are of particular interest when it comes to weight management, and this aspect is central to the Sirtfood Diet. Here's how sirtuins can impact weight and metabolism:

- **Metabolic Boost:** Sirtuins, particularly SIRT1, can enhance mitochondrial function and increase the body's energy expenditure. This means that activating sirtuins might lead to a higher metabolic rate, potentially aiding in weight loss.

- **Fat Utilization:** Sirtuins play a role in promoting the utilization of stored fat for energy. By activating sirtuins, it is theorized that the body may become more efficient at burning fat, which can contribute to weight loss and fat loss.

- **Appetite Regulation:** Sirtuins may influence appetite and food intake by interacting with hormones like leptin and ghrelin. This can help regulate hunger and reduce overeating.

- **Improved Insulin Sensitivity:** Sirtuins can enhance insulin sensitivity, which is important for glucose regulation and can help prevent insulin resistance, a precursor to type 2 diabetes.

It's important to note that while the science behind sirtuins is intriguing and promising, much of the research has been conducted in animal models and cell cultures. The exact mechanisms and effects of sirtuins in humans are still being studied, and their role in weight management and longevity is a topic of ongoing research. Additionally, lifestyle factors like diet and exercise also play a critical role in metabolic health and overall well-being, and sirtuins are just one piece of the puzzle.

CHAPTER 4

Getting Started with the Sirtfood Diet

4.1 Preparing Mentally and Emotionally

Embarking on any dietary journey, including the Sirtfood Diet, often requires mental and emotional preparation. Here are some key considerations:

- **Educate Yourself:** Start by understanding the core principles of the Sirtfood Diet, as well as its potential benefits and challenges. Knowledge is empowering and can help you make informed decisions.

- **Assess Your Motivation:** Reflect on why you want to try the Sirtfood Diet. Are you primarily interested in weight loss, better health, or other specific goals? Understanding your motivations can help you stay committed.

- **Manage Expectations:** Keep in mind that no diet is a magic solution. The Sirtfood Diet may offer benefits, but it's not a guaranteed path to instant results. Be realistic about what you can achieve and the time it might take.

- **Seek Support:** Consider discussing your plans with friends or family members who can offer encouragement and understanding. You might also find online communities or support groups related to the Sirtfood Diet for additional guidance and motivation.

- **Embrace Flexibility:** Understand that dietary changes can be challenging. Allow yourself flexibility to adapt and make modifications to the diet as needed. It's okay to have occasional deviations from the plan.

4.2 Setting Realistic Goals

Setting clear and achievable goals is crucial when starting the Sirtfood Diet:

- **Specific Goals:** Define specific, measurable goals. For example, you might aim to lose a certain amount of weight, improve your energy levels, or reduce inflammation markers.

- **Realistic Expectations:** Ensure your goals are realistic and attainable within a reasonable timeframe. Rapid, extreme changes are often unsustainable and can lead to disappointment.

- **Short-Term and Long-Term Goals:** Consider both short-term and long-term objectives. Short-term goals can provide motivation and milestones along the way to your larger, long-term goals.

- **Health-Centered Goals:** Focus on health outcomes rather than just weight loss. The Sirtfood Diet aims to promote overall well-being, so your goals should reflect that.

- **Consult a Healthcare Professional:** If you have specific health concerns or medical conditions, consult with a healthcare professional to set appropriate and safe goals tailored to your individual needs.

4.3 Creating a Meal Plan

A well-structured meal plan is essential for success on the Sirtfood Diet:

- **Identify Sirtfoods:** Start by identifying the Sirtfoods you enjoy and want to incorporate into your meals. Create a list of these foods to form the foundation of your plan.

- **Balanced Diet:** Ensure your meal plan includes a variety of Sirtfoods, along with other nutrient-rich foods to provide a balanced and complete diet. Incorporate lean proteins, whole grains, fruits, and vegetables.

- **Meal Timing:** Consider when you'll eat your meals and snacks. Some variations of the Sirtfood Diet emphasize intermittent fasting, while others encourage regular meals throughout the day. Choose an approach that suits your lifestyle.

- **Portion Control:** Pay attention to portion sizes to manage calorie intake. Even healthy foods can contribute to weight gain if consumed in excess.

- **Meal Preparation:** Plan and prepare your meals in advance to make it easier to stick to the diet. Prepping Sirtfood-rich dishes and snacks can help you avoid unhealthy choices when you're hungry.

- **Hydration:** Don't forget to stay hydrated by drinking water throughout the day. You can also include beverages like green tea, which is a Sirtfood.

- **Consult a Dietitian:** If you're unsure about creating a balanced meal plan or need personalized guidance, consider consulting a registered dietitian. They can help you design a meal plan tailored to your dietary preferences and health goals.

Sirtfood Diet is not one-size-fits-all, and individual needs and preferences vary. Your meal plan should be adaptable and sustainable for your specific lifestyle and goals. Additionally, it's important to monitor your progress and adjust your plan as needed to ensure it aligns with your evolving health and well-being.

CHAPTER 5

Phase 1: The Sirtfood Diet Jumpstart

Phase 1 of the Sirtfood Diet, often referred to as the "jumpstart" phase, is an initial period of more strict dietary adherence designed to kickstart your metabolism and potentially promote weight loss. Here's what you need to know:

5.1 The First 3 Days

- **Calorie Restriction:** During the first three days of the jumpstart phase, calorie intake is significantly restricted to around 1,000 to 1,500 calories per day. This calorie reduction is meant to create a calorie deficit, which can lead to weight loss.

- **Sirtfood Concentration:** Your meals in this phase will primarily consist of Sirtfoods. You'll be consuming Sirtfood-rich green juices and one balanced meal per day.

- **Green Juices:** You'll start your day with a green juice made from Sirtfoods. These juices are typically homemade and contain ingredients like kale, arugula, parsley, celery, green apple, lemon, and green tea. They are meant to be nutrient-dense and rich in sirtuin-activating compounds.

- **Balanced Meal:** Your one balanced meal should also include Sirtfoods. This can be a meal such as a Sirtfood salad with grilled chicken or fish. The emphasis is on a nutrient-dense, balanced meal that complements the Sirtfood-rich juices.

5.2 Sample Meal Plan

Here's a sample meal plan for one day during the first three days of the jumpstart phase:

Day 1:

Breakfast: Sirtfood Green Juice (kale, green apple, lemon, green tea)

Lunch: Sirtfood Green Juice

Dinner: Sirtfood Salad (kale, arugula, lovage, parsley, celery, walnuts, grilled chicken breast with olive oil and lemon dressing)

Note: Green tea and water can be consumed between meals to stay hydrated.

5.3 Tips for Success

Starting the Sirtfood Diet jumpstart phase can be challenging, but here are some tips to help you succeed:

- **Preparation is Key:** Plan your meals and green juices in advance. Prepare a shopping list and have all the necessary ingredients on hand.

- **Stay Hydrated:** Drink plenty of water and herbal teas throughout the day to stay hydrated. Green tea, which is a Sirtfood, can be a great choice.

- **Gradual Transition:** If you're not used to consuming green juices or following a lower-calorie diet, consider easing into the jumpstart phase by gradually reducing your calorie intake and increasing your consumption of Sirtfoods in the days leading up to it.

- **Listen to Your Body:** Pay attention to your body's signals. If you feel extremely fatigued or dizzy, it's important to reconsider whether the jumpstart phase is right for you or if you need to adjust the calorie restriction.

- **Seek Support:** Share your plan with a friend or family member for accountability and support. Having someone to discuss your experiences with can be motivating.

- **Consult a Healthcare Professional:** Before starting any restrictive diet, especially one as calorie-restricted as the jumpstart phase, it's wise to consult with a healthcare professional or registered dietitian to ensure it aligns with your health goals and needs.

It's important to remember that the jumpstart phase of the Sirtfood Diet is temporary and is followed by a more balanced and sustainable phase in which you continue to incorporate Sirtfoods into your daily meals. While the jumpstart phase may lead to initial weight loss, the long-term success of the diet depends on the ability to maintain a healthy and balanced diet over time.

CHAPTER 6

Phase 2: Maintenance and Sustainable Eating

After completing the initial jumpstart phase of the Sirtfood Diet, which is more restrictive in terms of calorie intake, many individuals transition into Phase 2. This phase is characterized by a more balanced and sustainable approach to eating. Here's what you need to know about transitioning to Phase 2:

6.1 Transitioning to Phase 2

Transitioning to Phase 2 of the Sirtfood Diet is an important step in maintaining the diet as a sustainable lifestyle. Here's how to make a smooth transition:

Gradual Calorie Increase: In Phase 2, you'll gradually increase your calorie intake compared to the jumpstart phase. This transition is crucial to prevent rapid weight regain and metabolic adaptations that can occur with extreme calorie restriction.

Diverse Food Choices: Phase 2 allows for a wider variety of foods beyond the Sirtfoods emphasized in the jumpstart phase. You'll still include Sirtfoods in your meals but also incorporate other nutrient-dense options to ensure a balanced diet.

Regular Meal Patterns: Establish regular eating patterns that suit your lifestyle. Some people find success with three meals a day, while others prefer smaller, more frequent meals. Find what works best for you and helps you maintain your desired calorie intake.

Portion Control: Continue to pay attention to portion sizes to manage calorie intake and avoid overeating. Maintaining portion control is key to successful weight management.

Mindful Eating: Practice mindful eating by being present during meals, savoring the flavors, and paying attention to hunger and fullness cues. This can help prevent mindless eating and emotional eating.

Long-Term Goals: Consider your long-term health goals. The Sirtfood

Diet is not just about short-term weight loss but also about supporting overall well-being. Focus on the health benefits of a balanced diet rich in Sirtfoods.

Variety and Balance: Embrace a wide variety of Sirtfoods and non-Sirtfoods to ensure a balanced and nutrient-rich diet. Include fruits, vegetables, lean proteins, whole grains, and healthy fats.

Stay Active: Continue to incorporate regular physical activity into your routine. Exercise complements the diet by supporting metabolic health and overall fitness.

Consult a Dietitian: If you have questions about transitioning to Phase 2 or need personalized guidance on meal planning, consider consulting a registered dietitian. They can help you create a sustainable and balanced eating plan that aligns with your specific dietary preferences and health goals.

Sirtfood Diet is meant to be a long-term lifestyle approach, not a short-term crash diet. Sustainability is key to reaping the potential health benefits of the diet. Phase 2 allows for more flexibility while still incorporating Sirtfoods into your meals, promoting metabolic health, and supporting your overall well-being.

6.2 Long-Term Sirtfood Eating

Long-term Sirtfood eating is the cornerstone of the Sirtfood Diet's sustainability and potential health benefits. To make Sirtfoods a permanent part of your dietary lifestyle, consider the following strategies:

- **Sirtfood Inclusion:** Continue to incorporate Sirtfoods into your meals regularly. These foods are rich in beneficial compounds and can contribute to your overall health and well-being.

- **Variety is Key:** Maintain variety in your diet by regularly rotating different Sirtfoods. This helps ensure that you receive a wide range of nutrients and phytochemicals.

- **Balanced Diet:** While Sirtfoods are important, remember that a balanced diet is essential for long-term health. Include a diverse range of foods, such as lean proteins, whole grains, fruits, and vegetables, to meet your nutritional needs.

- **Portion Control:** Keep an eye on portion sizes to maintain calorie balance. Overeating, even with healthy foods, can hinder your long-term goals.

- **Meal Planning:** Plan your meals in advance to ensure that you have Sirtfoods readily available. Having a structured meal plan makes it easier to maintain your dietary goals.

- **Mindful Eating:** Practice mindful eating by paying attention to hunger and fullness cues, and savoring the flavors of your food. This can help prevent overeating and promote a healthy relationship with food.

- **Regular Exercise:** Combine Sirtfood eating with regular physical activity. Exercise complements the diet by improving metabolism and overall health.

- **Consult a Dietitian:** If you have specific health goals or dietary concerns, consult a registered dietitian. They can help you create a customized long-term eating plan that incorporates Sirtfoods and aligns with your individual needs.

6.3 Recipe Ideas and Inspiration

To maintain long-term Sirtfood eating, you'll want a variety of delicious and nutritious recipes to keep your meals interesting. Here are some recipe ideas and sources of inspiration:

- **Sirtfood Salad:** Create a nutrient-packed salad with kale, arugula, parsley, celery, walnuts, and a dressing made from extra-virgin olive oil and lemon juice. Add grilled chicken, salmon, or tofu for protein.

- **Sirtfood Smoothies:** Blend Sirtfood-rich ingredients like kale, green apple, lemon, and green tea into smoothies. You can customize these by adding

Greek yogurt, berries, or
protein powder.

- **Sirtfood Stir-Fry:** Prepare a
stir-fry with Sirtfoods like
broccoli, bok choy, and green
beans. Add lean protein sources
like chicken or shrimp, and use
a sauce made with garlic,
ginger, and soy sauce.

- **Sirtfood Omelette:** Make a
Sirtfood omelette with eggs,
kale, red onions, and tomatoes.
Top it with grated Parmesan
cheese for added flavor.

- **Sirtfood Soup:** Prepare a
Sirtfood soup by blending
vegetables like kale, spinach,
and onions with vegetable or
chicken broth. Add beans for
extra protein and fiber.

- **Sirtfood Curry:** Create a Sirtfood-rich curry using ingredients like turmeric, garlic, ginger, and green tea. Add vegetables and your choice of protein, such as chicken, tofu, or lentils.

- **Sirtfood Smoothie Bowl:** Turn your Sirtfood smoothie into a bowl by adding toppings like sliced bananas, chia seeds, and chopped nuts for added texture and flavor.

- **Online Resources:** Explore Sirtfood recipe websites, cookbooks, and social media platforms where individuals share their Sirtfood meal creations for inspiration and new ideas.

The key to long-term Sirtfood eating is to make it enjoyable and sustainable. Experiment with recipes, adapt them to your taste preferences, and find joy in preparing and sharing Sirtfood-rich meals with friends and family.

CHAPTER 7

Sirtfood Diet and Weight Loss

7.1 How the Diet Supports Weight Loss

The Sirtfood Diet is often associated with weight loss due to several key mechanisms and principles that support this goal:

1. **Calorie Restriction:** During the initial phase of the Sirtfood Diet, the jumpstart phase, there is a significant reduction in calorie intake. This calorie deficit is achieved by consuming green juices and a balanced meal that is lower in

calories. A calorie deficit is a fundamental factor in weight loss, as it encourages the body to use stored fat for energy.

2. **Metabolic Boost:** Sirtfoods, particularly those rich in resveratrol, such as red wine, can potentially increase metabolic rate. When metabolism is higher, the body burns more calories at rest, making it easier to lose weight.

3. **Fat Utilization:** The diet emphasizes the consumption of foods that may enhance the body's ability to use stored fat as an energy source. This is especially true during the jumpstart phase, which can contribute to fat loss.

4. **Appetite Regulation:** Sirtfoods have been suggested to help regulate appetite. By including them in your meals, you may feel fuller for longer, reducing the likelihood of overeating or snacking between meals.

5. **Muscle Preservation:** The Sirtfood Diet promotes the preservation of lean muscle mass, as it includes sufficient protein intake. Preserving muscle mass is crucial during weight loss to maintain metabolic rate and support overall body composition.

6. **Anti-Inflammatory Effects:** Chronic inflammation can contribute to weight gain and obesity-related complications. Sirtfoods, with their potential anti-inflammatory properties,

may help reduce inflammation, which can support weight loss efforts.

7. **Balanced Nutrition:** While the jumpstart phase of the Sirtfood Diet is calorie-restricted, Phase 2 emphasizes balanced nutrition. This ensures that you still receive essential nutrients, making it easier to maintain a healthy eating pattern over time.

8. **Improved Insulin Sensitivity:** Sirtuins, activated by Sirtfoods, are associated with improved insulin sensitivity. Enhanced insulin sensitivity can help regulate blood sugar levels and prevent the excessive storage of glucose as fat.

9. **Long-Term Lifestyle Approach:** The Sirtfood Diet promotes a long-term lifestyle approach to eating, rather than a short-term crash diet. This sustainable approach is more likely to lead to gradual, lasting weight loss and maintenance.

It's important to note that while the Sirtfood Diet may offer weight loss benefits, individual results can vary. Success in losing and maintaining weight depends on factors such as adherence to the diet, overall calorie intake, physical activity level, genetics, and individual metabolic rate. Additionally, the Sirtfood Diet should be followed with consideration of individual health goals and needs, and it may not be suitable for everyone. Consulting with a healthcare professional or registered dietitian before starting any new diet plan is advisable, especially if you have underlying health conditions or specific weight loss goals.

7.2 Realistic Expectations

When embarking on the Sirtfood Diet or any weight loss journey, it's important to have realistic expectations. Here's what you should keep in mind:

1. **Gradual Progress:** Sustainable weight loss typically occurs gradually, at a rate of about 0.5 to 2 pounds (0.2 to 0.9 kilograms) per week. Rapid or extreme weight loss is often unsustainable and can lead to health issues.

2. **Individual Variation:** Weight loss results can vary widely from person to person. Factors such as genetics, metabolism, starting weight, and lifestyle play significant roles in determining how quickly and how much weight you can lose.

3. **Plateaus:** Weight loss is not always linear. It's common to experience periods of plateau, where your weight remains stable despite your efforts. This is normal and doesn't necessarily mean the diet isn't working.

4. **Health Benefits Beyond Weight Loss:** Remember that the Sirtfood Diet promotes overall health and well-being, not just weight loss. Focus on the broader benefits, such as

improved metabolic health and reduced inflammation.

5. **Sustainability:** A diet that is too restrictive or difficult to maintain in the long term is unlikely to lead to lasting weight loss. The Sirtfood Diet encourages a sustainable approach to eating that you can continue over time.

6. **Health-Centered Goals:** Consider setting health-centered goals alongside weight loss goals. These could include improved energy levels, better blood sugar control, reduced inflammation, or enhanced overall fitness.

7. **Consult a Professional:** If you have specific weight loss goals or health concerns, consult with

a healthcare professional or registered dietitian. They can help you set realistic and individualized goals based on your unique circumstances.

7.3 Monitoring Progress

Monitoring your progress while following the Sirtfood Diet or any weight loss plan is important for staying on track and making necessary adjustments. Here's how you can effectively monitor your progress:

1. **Regular Weigh-Ins:** Weigh yourself consistently, such as once a week, at the same time of day and under the same conditions (e.g., in the morning after using the bathroom and before eating). Keep a record of

your weight to track changes over time.

2. **Body Measurements:** In addition to weight, measure key body areas such as your waist, hips, and thighs. Changes in measurements can provide insights into your progress, especially when the scale may not reflect changes accurately.

3. **Progress Photos:** Take before-and-after photos to visually track changes in your physique. These photos can be motivating and help you see changes that may not be immediately evident on the scale.

4. **Energy Levels:** Pay attention to changes in your energy levels and overall well-being. Improved energy and mood can

be signs of progress, even if weight loss is gradual.

5. **Clothing Fit:** Notice how your clothes fit. Changes in clothing size or comfort can be a positive indicator of progress.

6. **Physical Performance:** Assess changes in physical performance, such as increased stamina during workouts, improved strength, or enhanced flexibility. These improvements indicate increased fitness levels.

7. **Non-Scale Victories:** Celebrate non-scale victories, such as better sleep, reduced cravings, improved digestion, or reduced inflammation markers. These changes contribute to overall well-being.

8. **Consult a Professional:** If
    you're uncertain about your
    progress or how to effectively
    track it, consult with a
    healthcare professional or
    registered dietitian. They can
    provide guidance on the most
    appropriate metrics for your
    individual goals and help you
    interpret your results.

progress may not always be linear, and there will be fluctuations along the way. Focus on the positive changes you're experiencing, and use the information you gather to make informed decisions about your dietary and lifestyle choices. Additionally, weight management should always be approached with a focus on overall health, not just the number on the scale.

CHAPTER 8

Incorporating Exercise and Lifestyle Changes

Incorporating exercise and lifestyle changes alongside a healthy diet like the Sirtfood Diet can enhance overall well-being and support your health and fitness goals. Here's how to approach exercise and lifestyle adjustments:

8.1 The Role of Exercise

Exercise plays a crucial role in promoting overall health, weight management, and fitness. When combined with a balanced diet like the Sirtfood Diet, exercise can be even more effective. Here are some key points to consider:

- **Aerobic Exercise:** Engage in regular aerobic exercise, such as brisk walking, jogging, swimming, or cycling. Aerobic activities help burn calories, improve cardiovascular health, and enhance endurance.

- **Strength Training:** Incorporate strength training exercises, such as weightlifting or bodyweight exercises, to build and maintain lean muscle mass. Muscle burns more calories at rest than fat, contributing to a higher metabolic rate.

- **Flexibility and Mobility:**
  Include flexibility and mobility
  exercises, such as yoga or
  stretching routines, to improve
  joint health and reduce the risk
  of injury.

- **Regularity is Key:** Aim for
  consistency in your exercise
  routine. Establish a regular
  schedule that includes both
  aerobic and strength training
  exercises.

- **Progressive Overload:**
  Gradually increase the intensity
  and duration of your workouts
  as your fitness level improves.
  This helps prevent plateaus and
  promotes continuous
  improvement.

- **Consult a Fitness
  Professional:** If you're new to

exercise or have specific fitness goals, consider consulting a fitness professional, such as a personal trainer or physical therapist. They can create a customized exercise plan tailored to your needs.

- **Listen to Your Body:** Pay attention to your body's signals and avoid overtraining or pushing yourself too hard. Adequate rest and recovery are essential for preventing burnout and injuries.

8.2 Stress Management and Sleep

Stress management and quality sleep are integral components of a healthy lifestyle that complement dietary and exercise efforts:

- **Stress Reduction:** Chronic stress can lead to weight gain and disrupt healthy eating patterns. Incorporate stress-reduction techniques such as meditation, deep breathing exercises, mindfulness, or hobbies that bring joy and relaxation into your life.

- **Adequate Sleep:** Prioritize sleep as a fundamental aspect of health. Aim for 7-9 hours of quality sleep per night. Lack of sleep can disrupt hormones that regulate appetite and lead to overeating.

- **Bedtime Routine:** Create a bedtime routine that signals to your body that it's time to wind down. Avoid screens before bed, keep the bedroom cool and dark, and establish a consistent sleep schedule.

- **Limit Caffeine and Alcohol:** Reduce caffeine and alcohol consumption, especially in the evening, as they can interfere with sleep quality.

8.3 Staying Active and Healthy

Maintaining an active and healthy lifestyle goes beyond structured exercise and sleep management. Here are additional tips to help you stay on track:

- **Hydration:** Drink plenty of water throughout the day to stay hydrated. Proper hydration supports overall health and can help control appetite.

- **Mindful Eating:** Continue practicing mindful eating by being present during meals and paying attention to hunger and fullness cues. Avoid distracted eating, which can lead to overconsumption.

- **Social Support:** Share your health and fitness goals with friends or family members who can provide encouragement and accountability. Consider joining fitness classes or groups in your community for added support.

- **Limit Processed Foods:** Minimize the consumption of processed and sugary foods, as they can contribute to weight

gain and health issues. Focus
on whole, nutrient-dense foods.

- **Regular Health Checkups:**
  Schedule regular checkups with
  your healthcare provider to
  monitor your overall health,
  including blood pressure,
  cholesterol levels, and other
  key indicators.

- **Set Realistic Goals:**
  Continuously set realistic and
  achievable goals for your health
  and fitness journey. Celebrate
  your successes along the way,
  no matter how small.

- **Adaptability:** Be adaptable
  and flexible in your approach.
  Life may present challenges
  and disruptions, but the key is
  to find ways to get back on

track and stay committed to
your long-term health goals.

holistic approach to health and fitness
is essential. While the Sirtfood Diet
can provide dietary guidelines,
incorporating exercise, stress
management, and healthy lifestyle
habits will contribute to a well-
rounded and sustainable approach to
overall well-being.

CHAPTER 9

Common Challenges and How to Overcome Them

Navigating the Sirtfood Diet or any dietary plan can come with its share of challenges. Here's how to address some common challenges and overcome them:

9.1 Dealing with Cravings

Cravings for unhealthy foods can be a hurdle in any diet. Here's how to manage cravings on the Sirtfood Diet:

- **Sirtfood Alternatives:** Identify Sirtfood-rich alternatives for your favorite cravings. For example, if you crave chocolate, opt for dark chocolate with a high cocoa content as it contains Sirtuin-activating compounds.

- **Mindful Eating:** When a craving strikes, pause and practice mindful eating. Ask yourself if you're truly hungry or if the craving is driven by emotions or boredom. Sometimes a glass of water or a

small Sirtfood-rich snack can
satisfy your craving.

- **Healthy Substitutes:**
Experiment with healthy
substitutes for unhealthy foods.
For instance, swap regular
potato chips for baked kale
chips or indulge in Sirtfood-
rich berries instead of sugary
desserts.

- **Portion Control:** If you give in
to a craving, practice portion
control. Enjoy a small amount
of the desired food rather than
indulging excessively.

- **Stay Hydrated:** Sometimes
dehydration can be mistaken
for hunger or cravings. Drink a
glass of water when cravings
strike to see if it subsides.

- **Distract Yourself:** Engage in an activity or hobby you enjoy when cravings are strong. Distraction can help redirect your focus away from food.

- **Plan for Treats:** Consider incorporating occasional treats into your diet to satisfy cravings in a controlled manner. Just be mindful of portion sizes and frequency.

9.2 Social and Dining Out Challenges

Maintaining the Sirtfood Diet in social settings and while dining out can be challenging, but it's manageable:

- **Plan Ahead:** When dining out, review the restaurant menu in advance if possible. Look for dishes that include Sirtfoods or can be customized to fit the diet.

- **Communicate:** Don't hesitate to communicate your dietary preferences and restrictions to the restaurant staff. Many restaurants are willing to accommodate special requests.

- **Choose Wisely:** opt for dishes that naturally align with the Sirtfood Diet, such as salads with Sirtfood-rich ingredients, grilled lean proteins, and vegetable-based dishes.

- **Control Portions:** Pay attention to portion sizes when dining out. Restaurant portions tend to be larger than what you might prepare at home, so consider sharing dishes or taking leftovers home.

- **BYO Snacks:** If you anticipate hunger between meals while socializing, bring Sirtfood-friendly snacks with you, such as a bag of kale chips or a small container of Sirtfood berries.

- **Enjoy in Moderation:** In social settings, it's okay to indulge occasionally, but practice moderation. Enjoy the company and the food but avoid overindulging.

9.3 Plateau Busting Strategies

Plateaus are common during weight loss efforts. Here's how to break through a weight loss plateau on the Sirtfood Diet:

- **Reevaluate Portions:** Assess your portion sizes and calorie intake. You may need to adjust your portion control to create a new calorie deficit.

- **Diversify Sirtfoods:** Introduce new Sirtfoods into your diet or rotate them to prevent metabolic adaptation. Experiment with different Sirtfood-rich recipes to keep your meals exciting.

- **Increase Exercise Intensity:** If you've reached a plateau, consider increasing the intensity or duration of your workouts to boost calorie expenditure.

- **Interval Training:** Incorporate interval training into your exercise routine. High-intensity interval training (HIIT) can help rev up your metabolism and break through plateaus.

- **Change Exercise Routine:** Alter your exercise routine by trying new activities or workouts. Your body can adapt to the same routine over time, leading to plateaus.

- **Stay Hydrated:** Ensure you're drinking enough water, as dehydration can slow down metabolism. Hydration is important for overall health and weight loss.

- **Consult a Professional:** If you've hit a persistent plateau, consider consulting a healthcare professional or registered dietitian. They can provide personalized guidance and assess whether underlying factors may be affecting your progress.

plateaus are a natural part of the weight loss journey. Be patient and persistent, and focus on overall health and well-being rather than just the number on the scale. Adjustments in your diet and exercise routine can help you overcome plateaus and continue progressing toward your goals.

www.ingramcontent.com/pod-product-compliance
Lightning Source LLC
Chambersburg PA
CBHW061001260726
48661CB00005B/1984